THE
40 MOST BEAUTIFUL
FLOWER GARDENS
IN THE WORLD

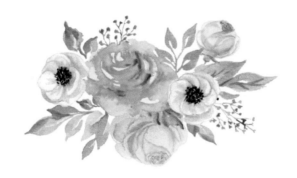

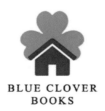

**BLUE CLOVER
BOOKS**

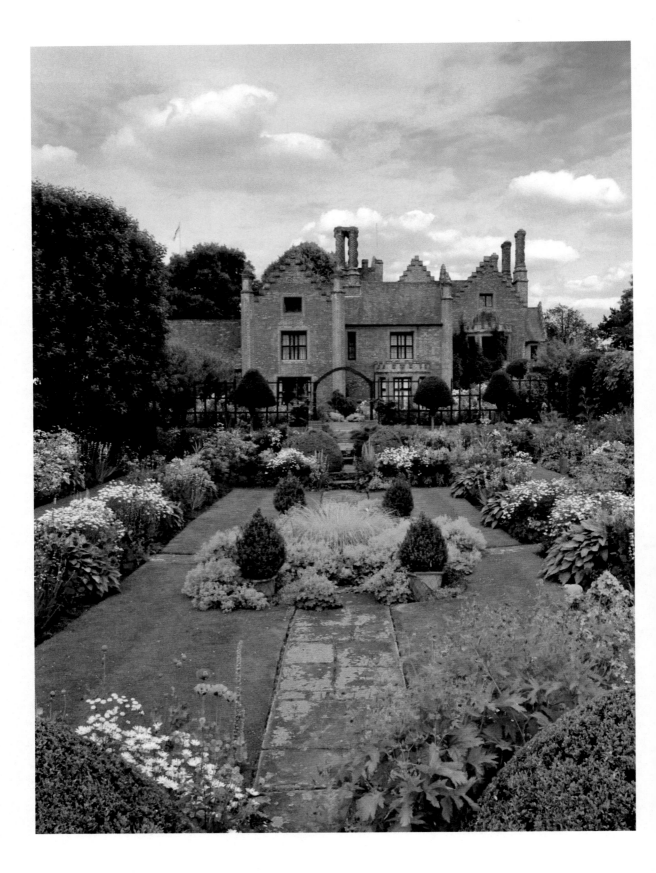

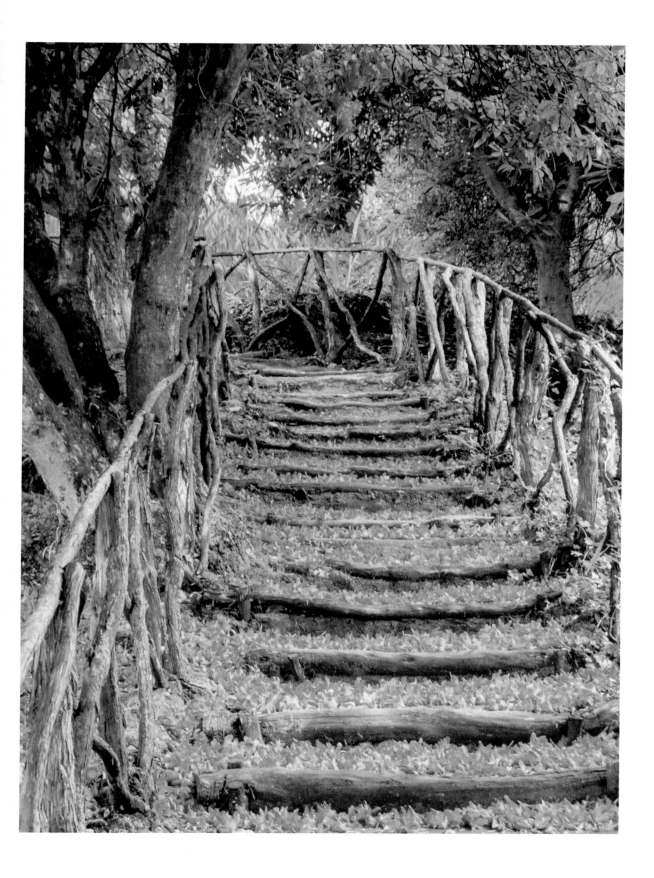

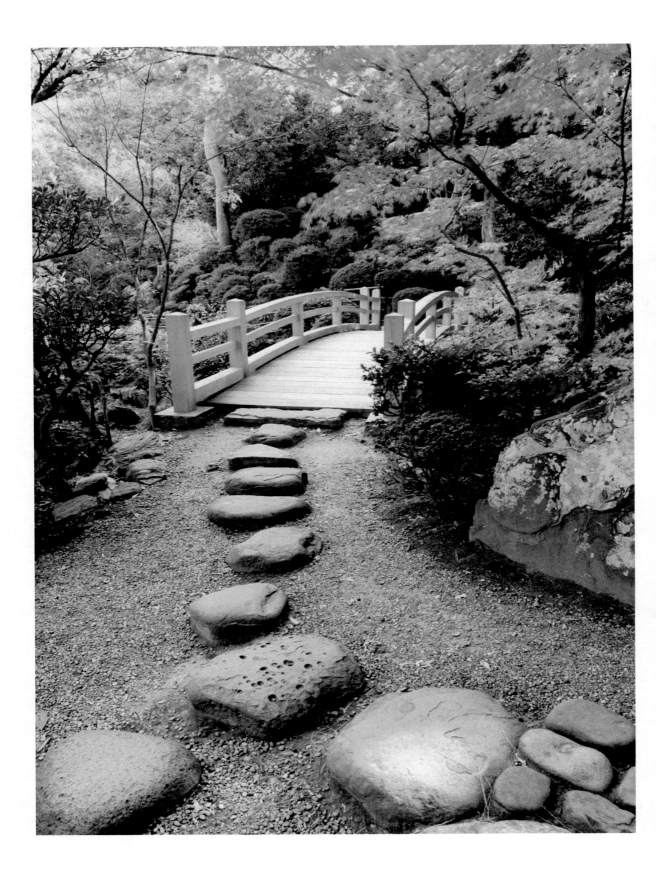

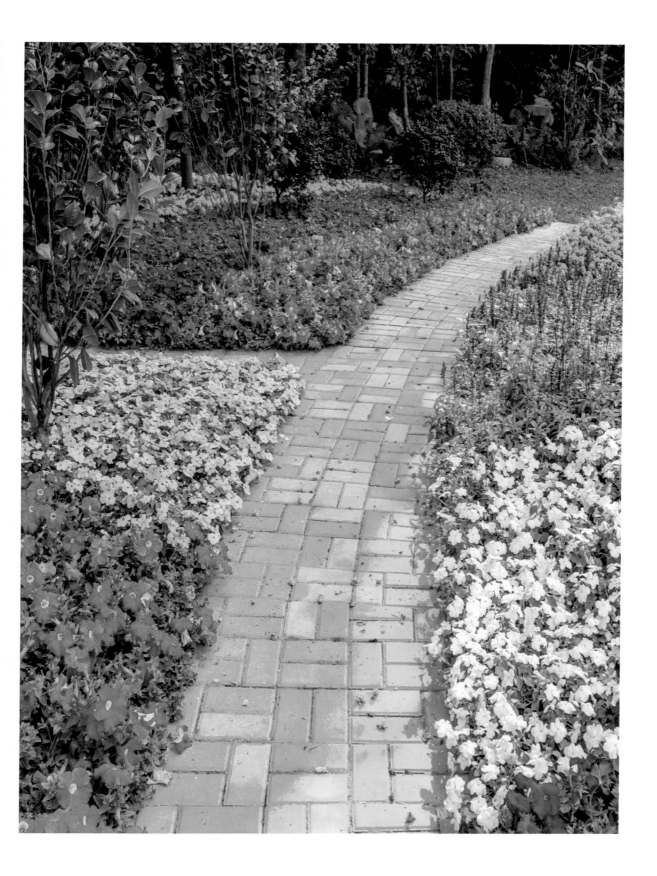

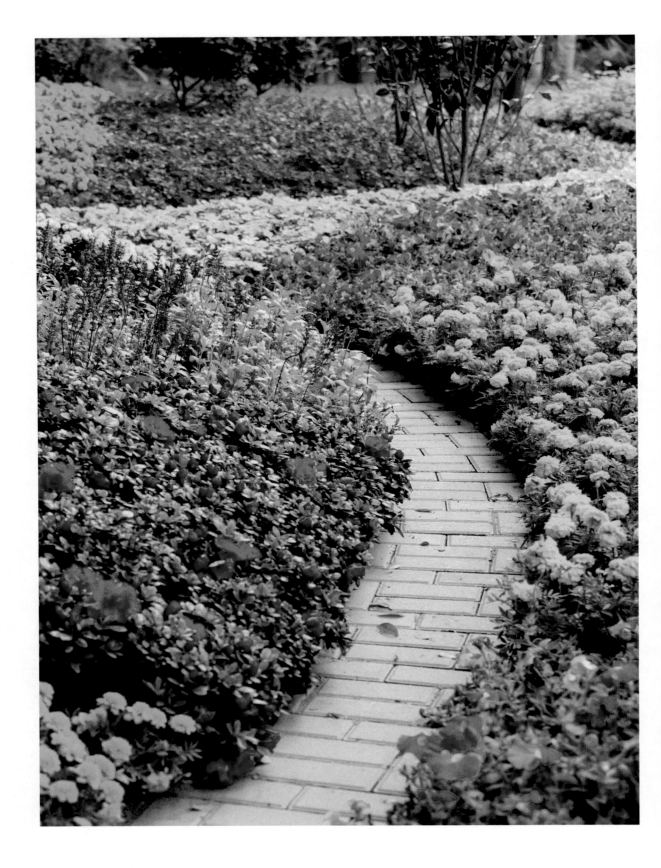

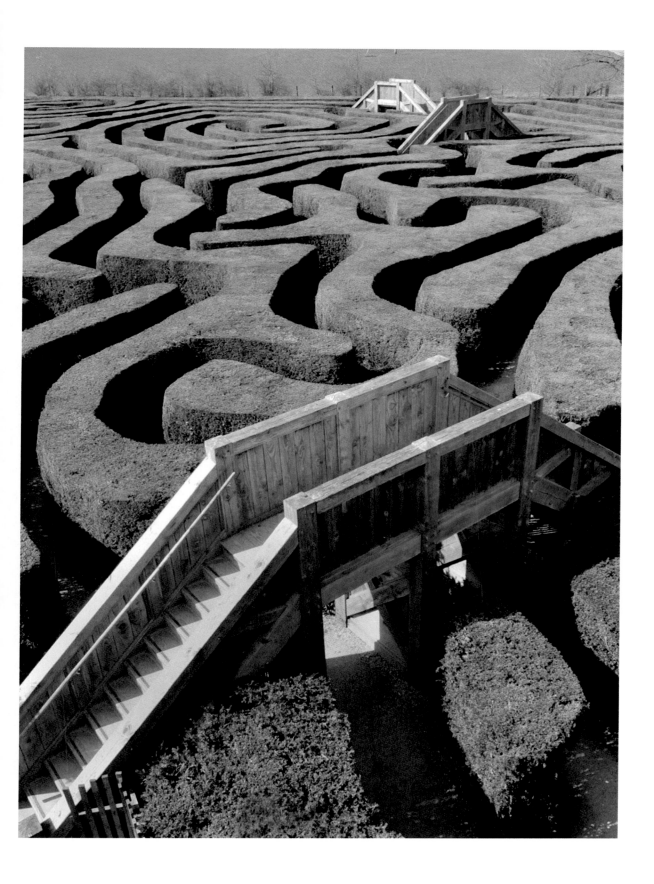

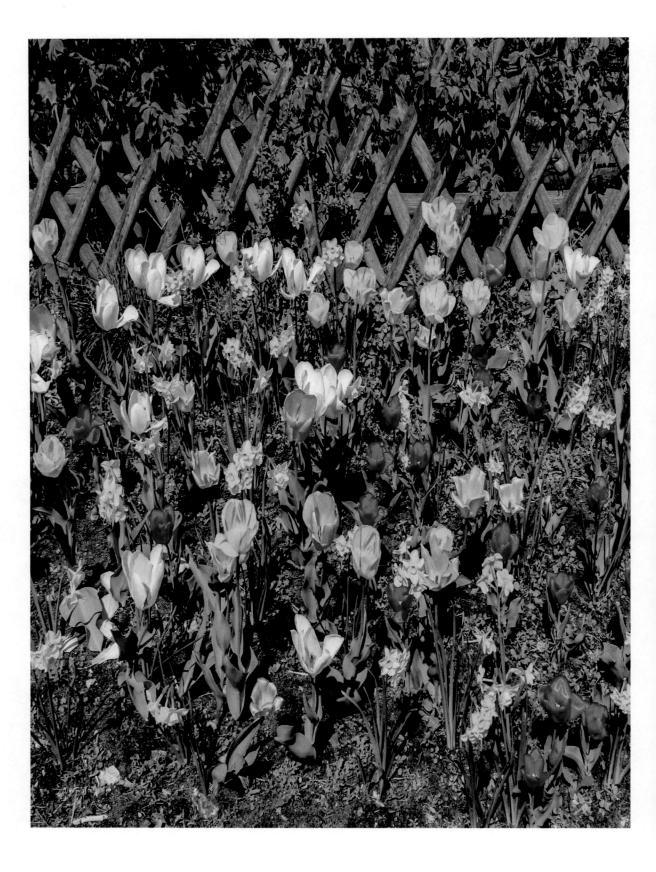

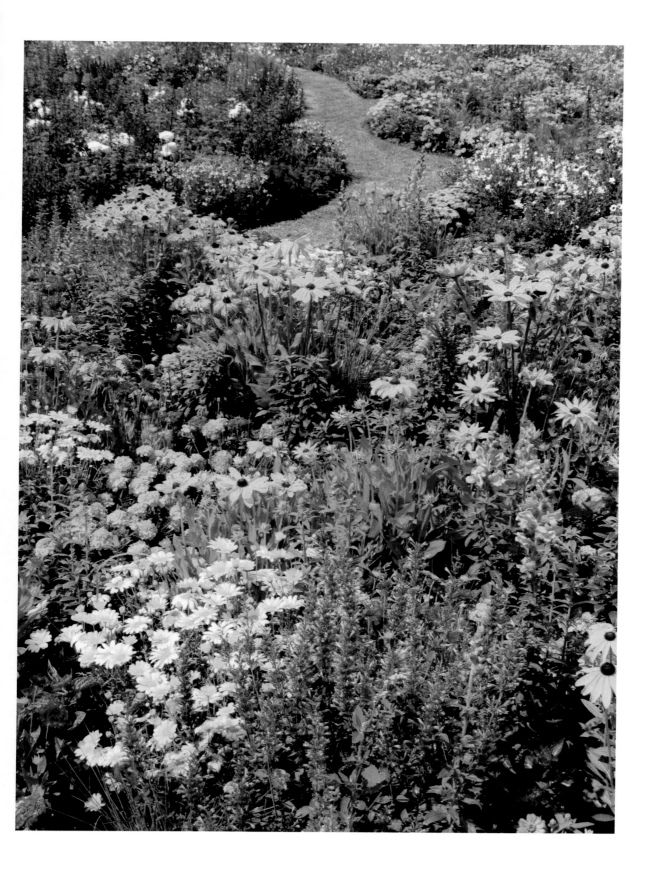

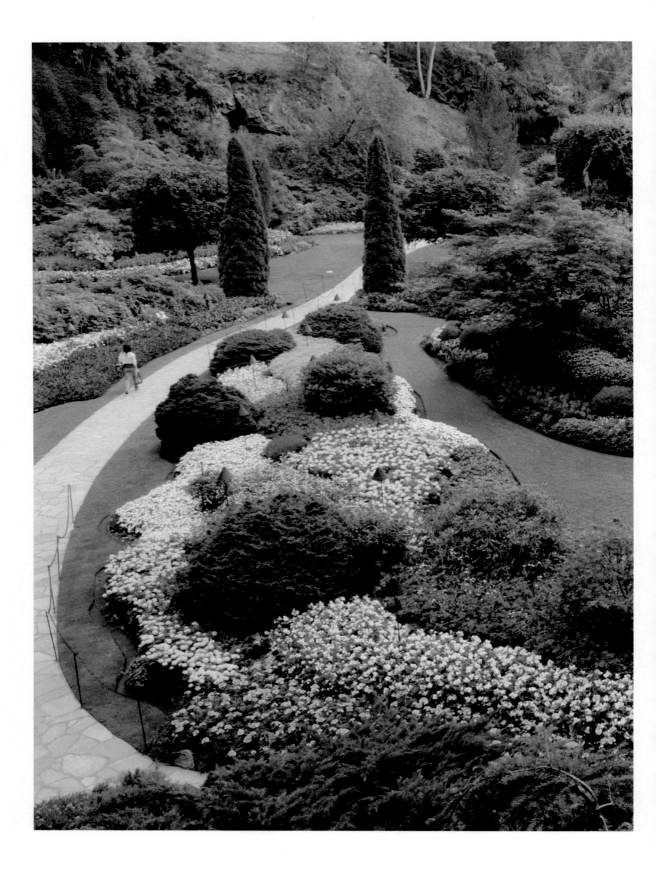

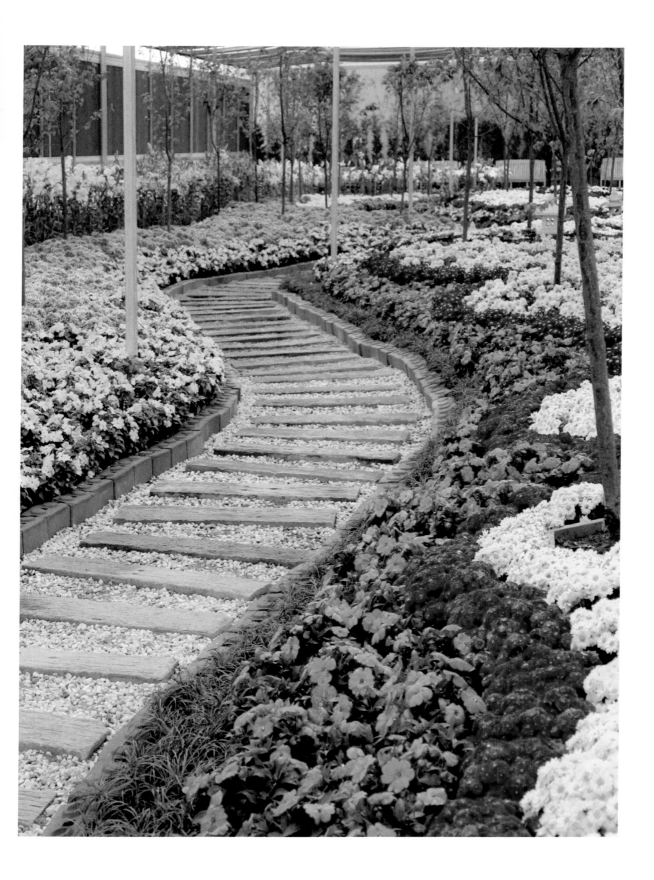

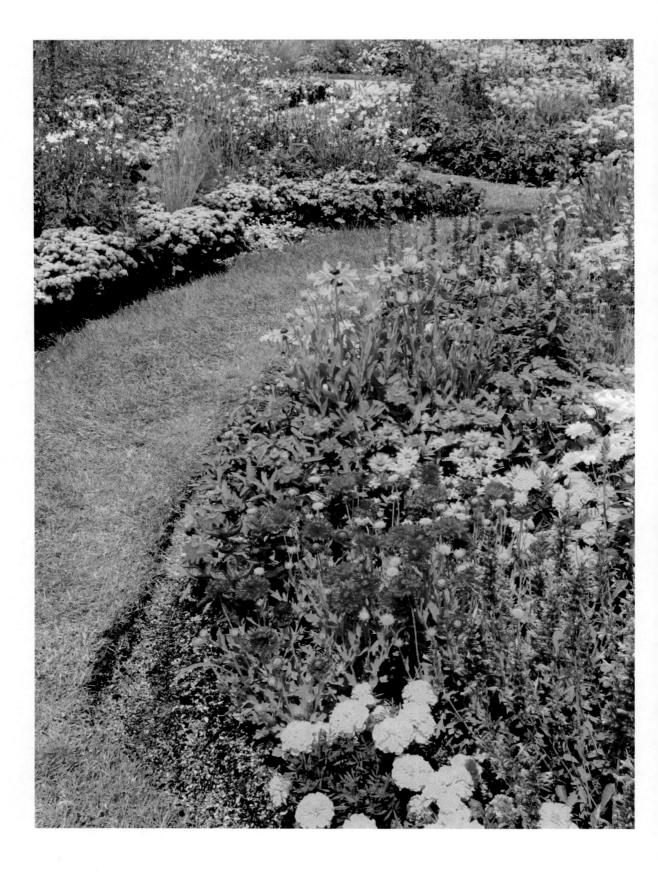

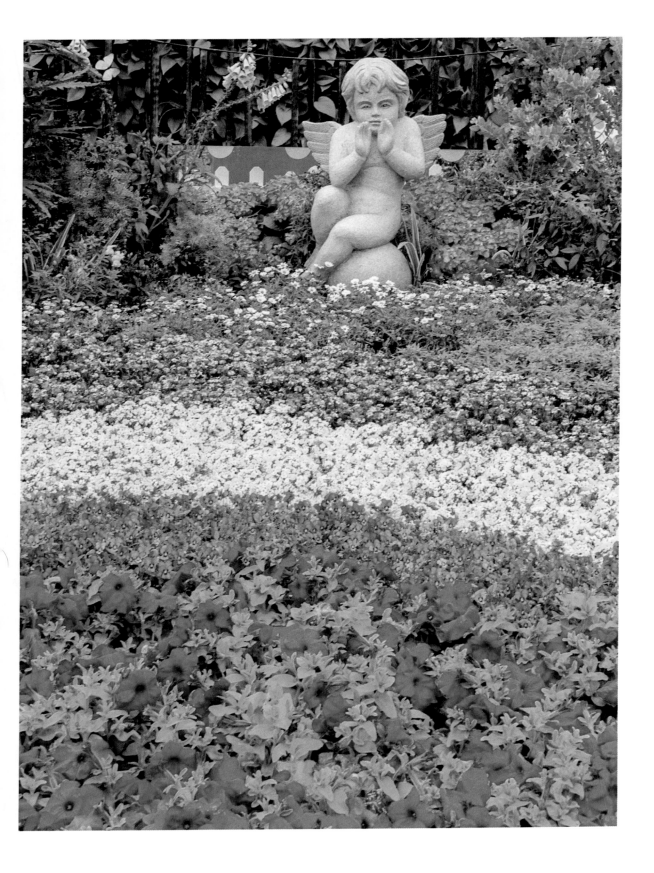

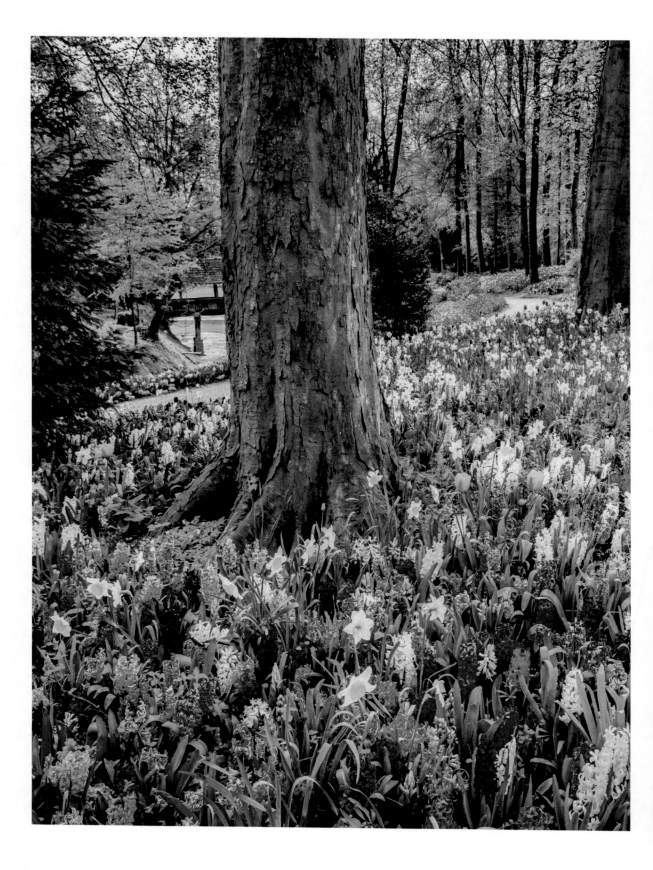

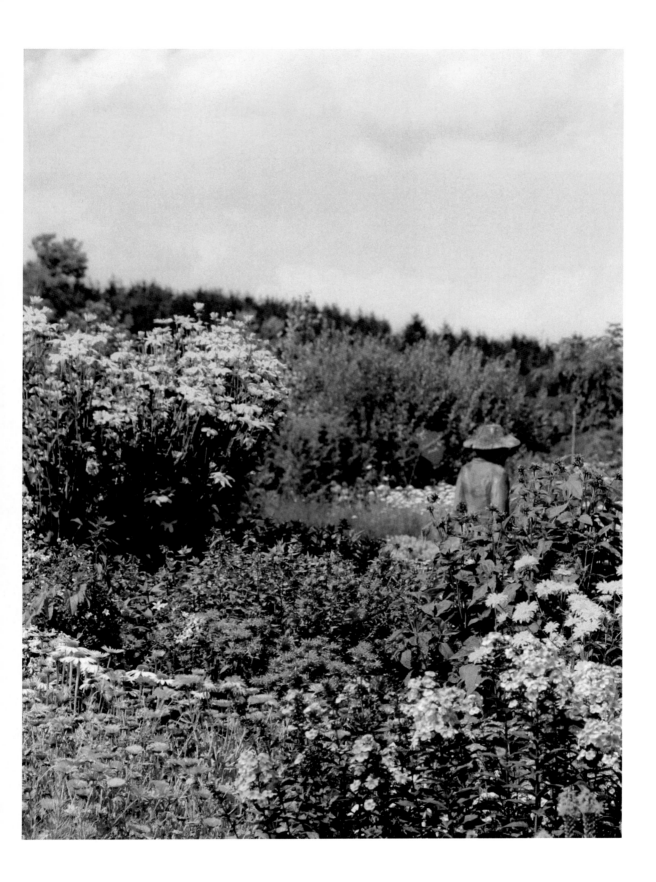

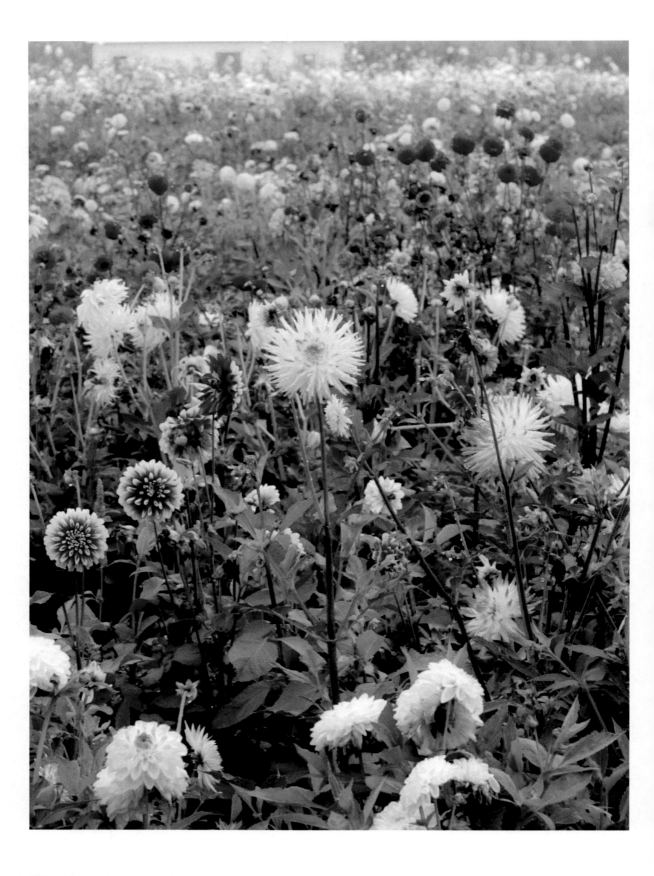

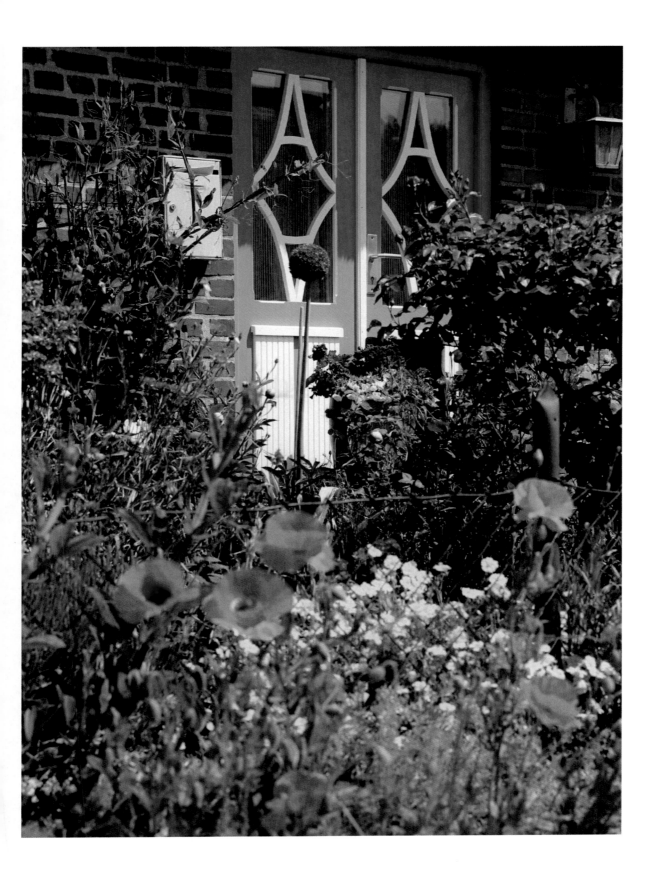

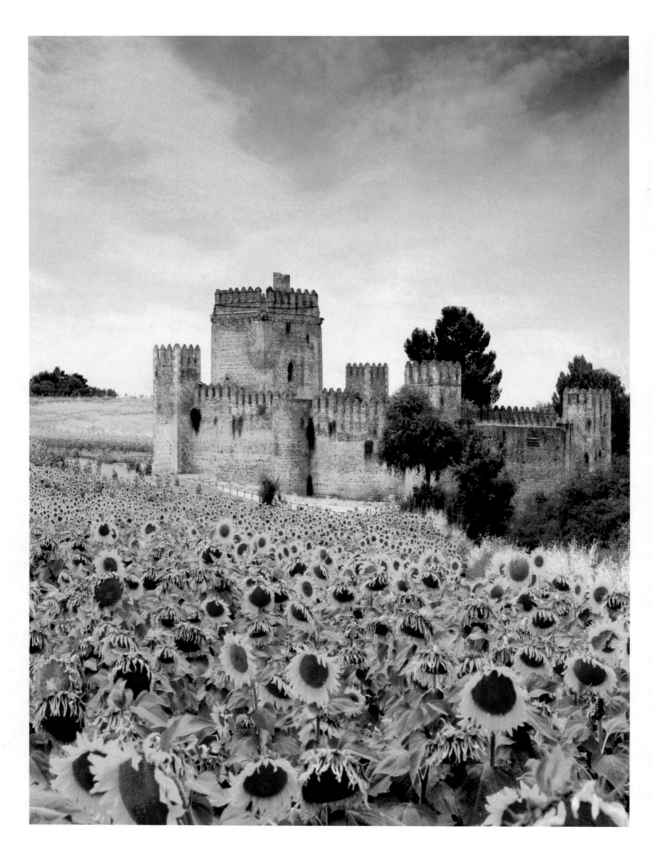

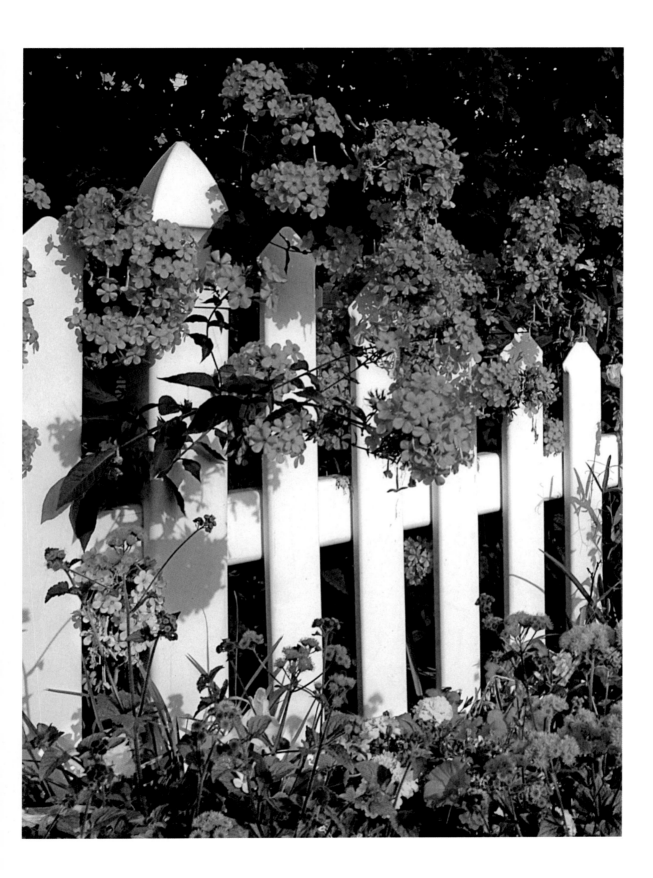

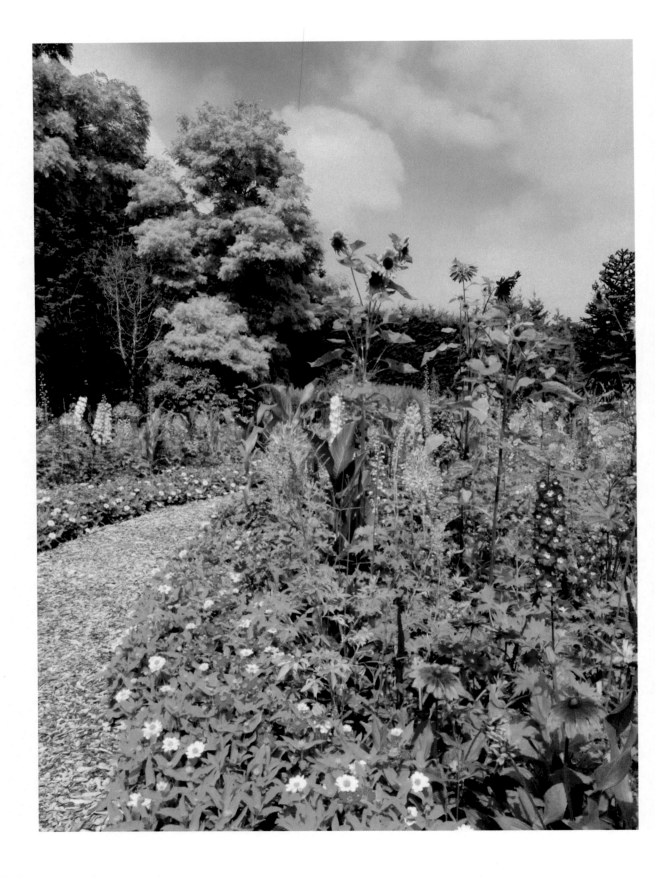

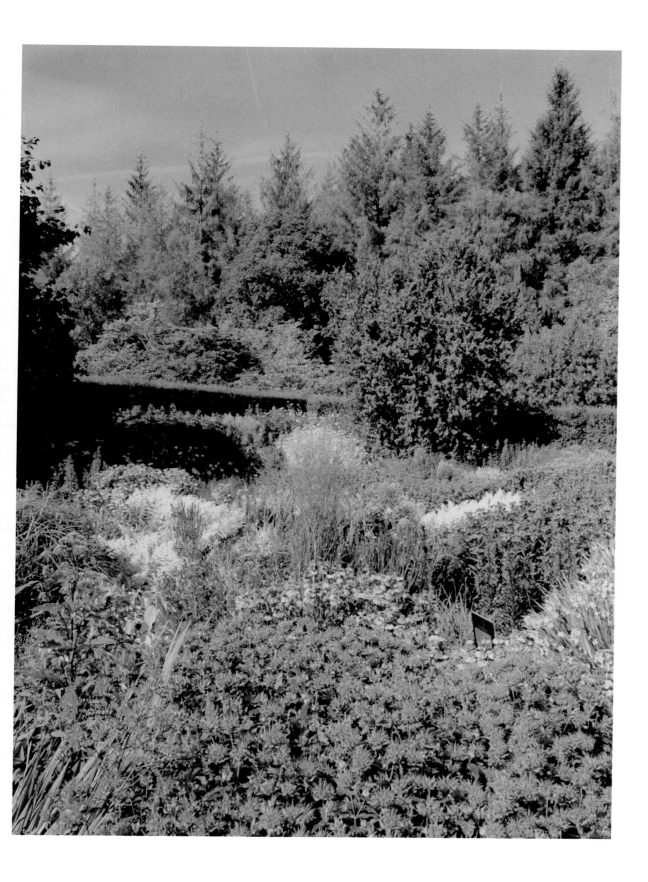

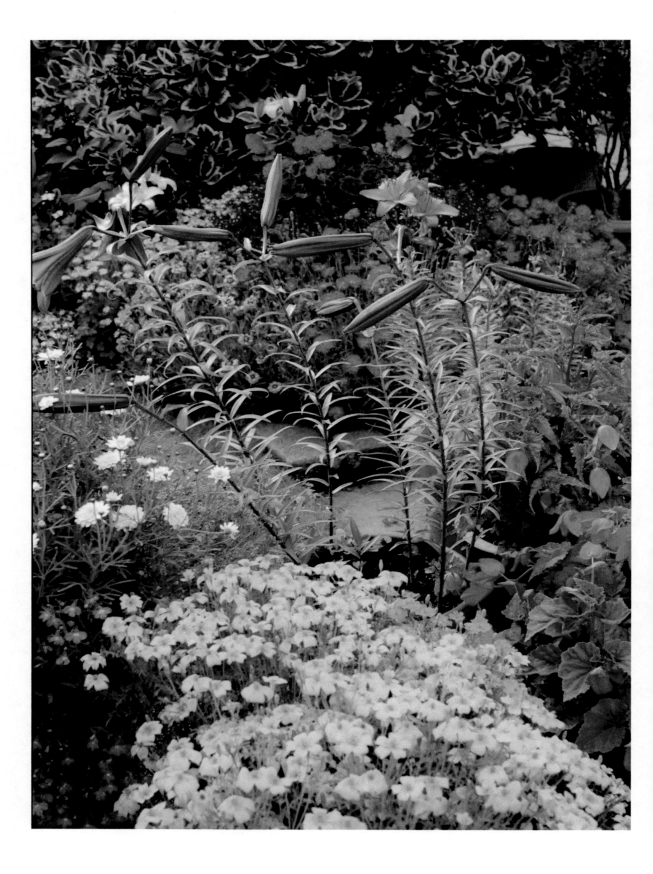

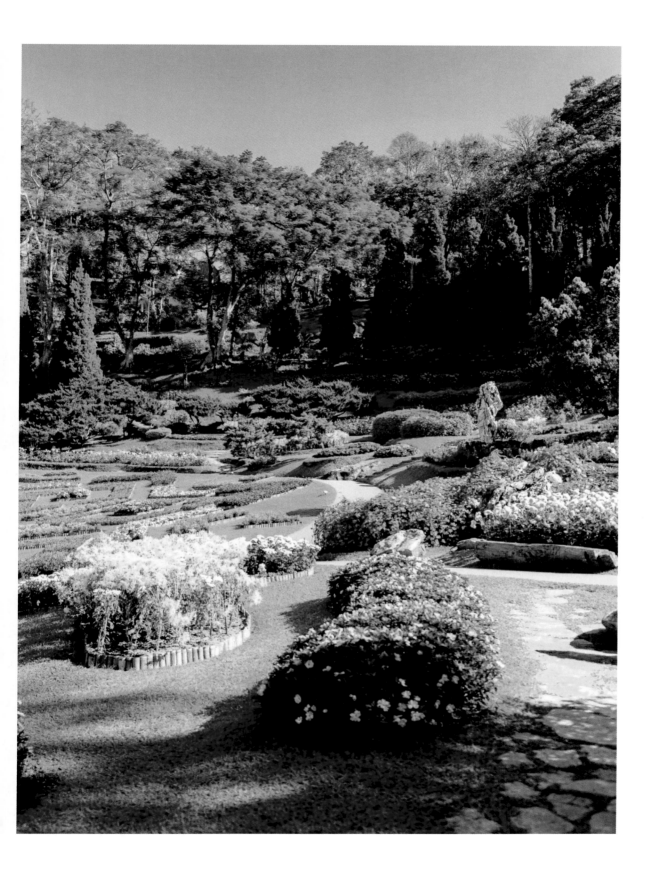

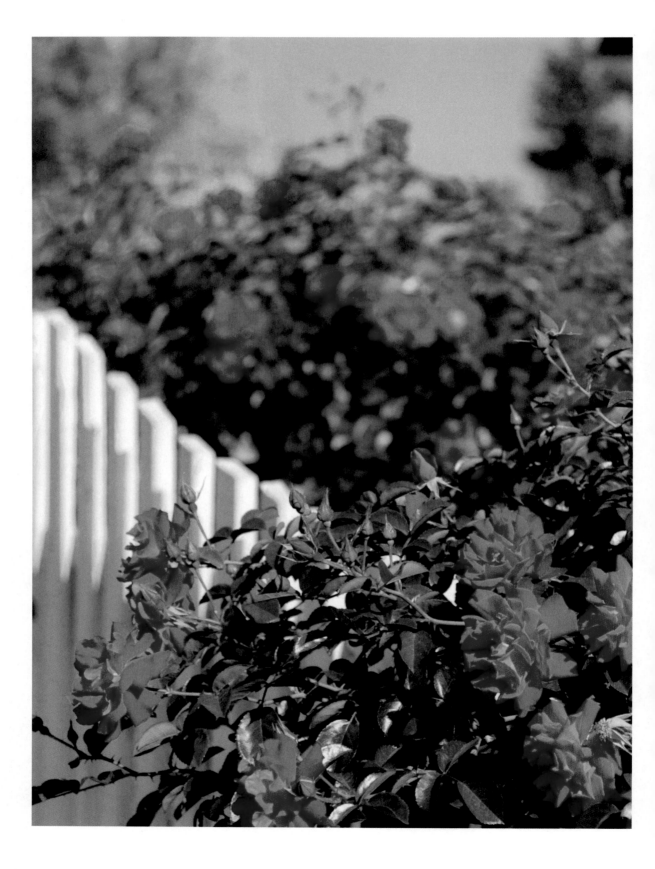

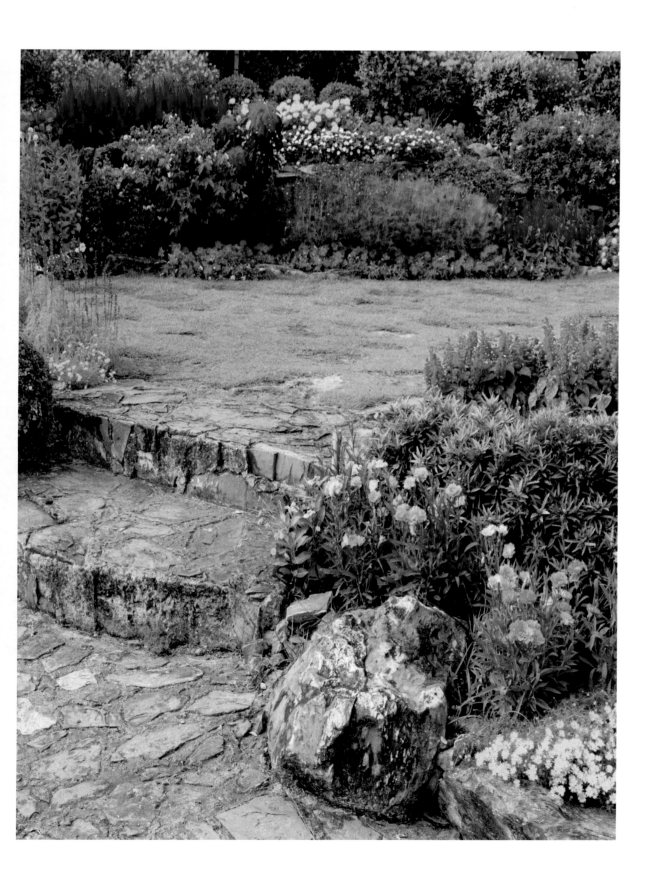

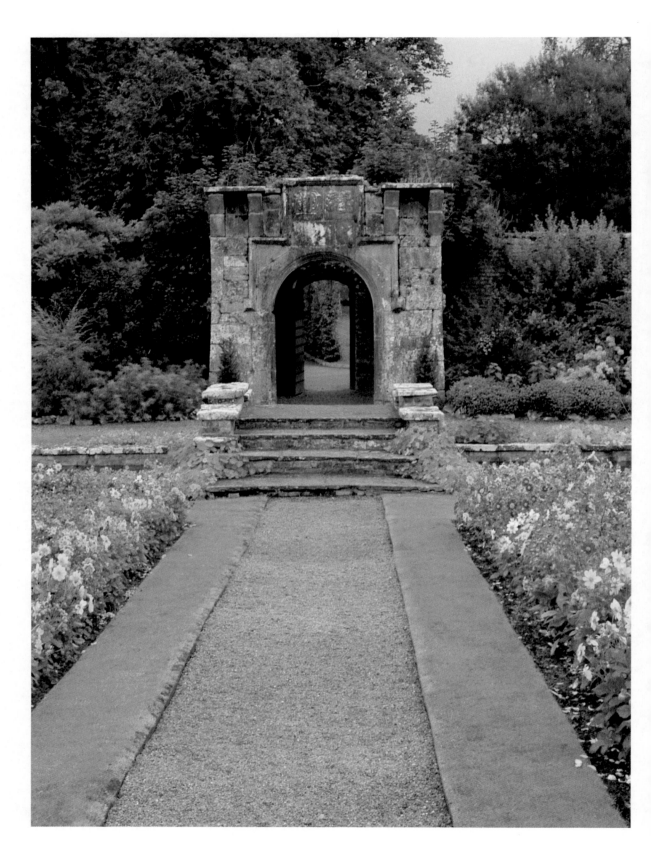

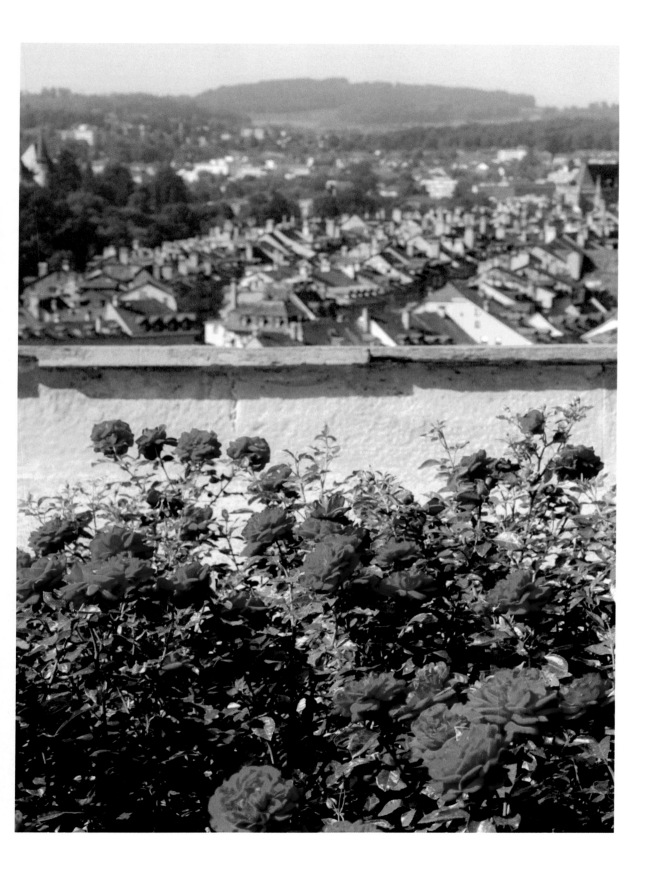

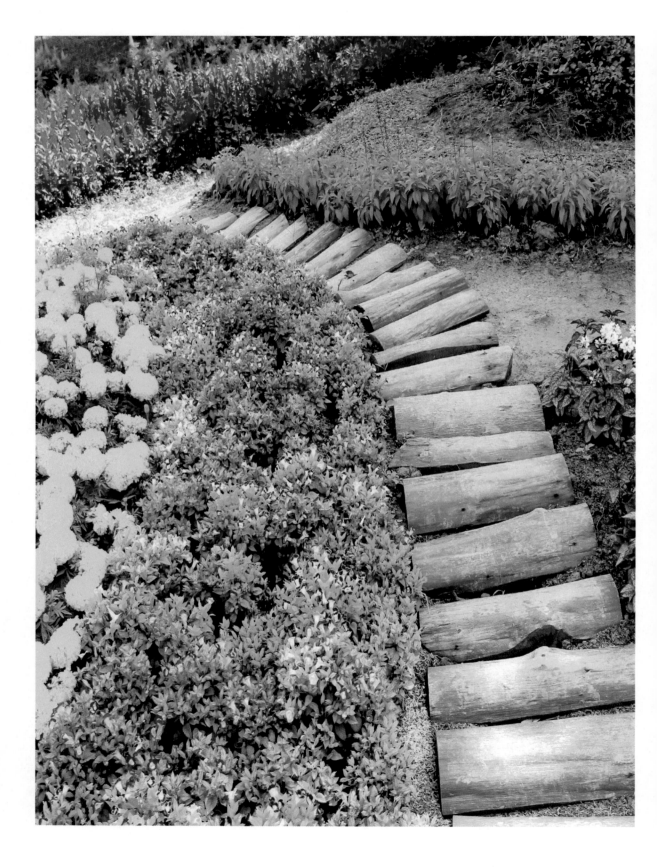

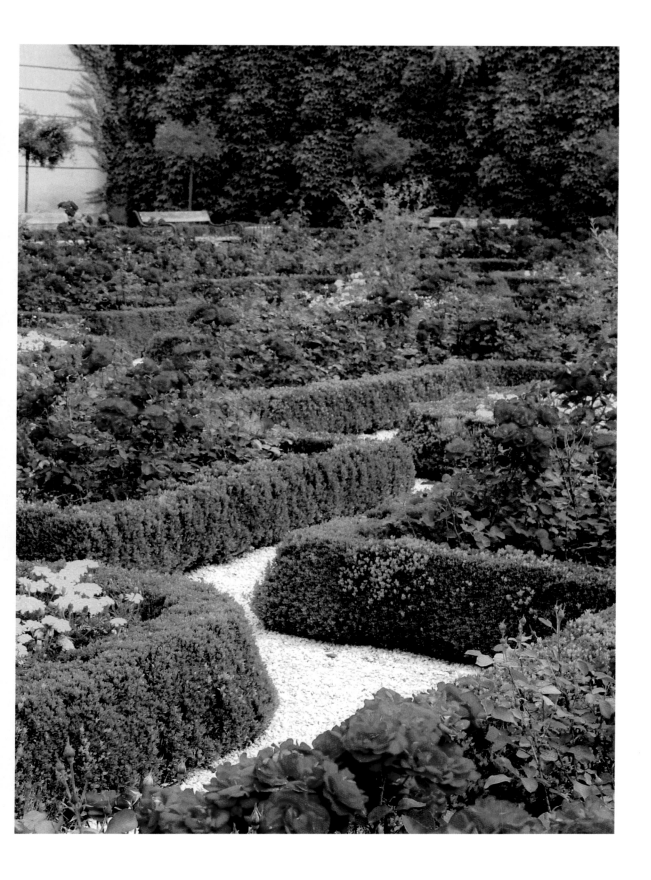

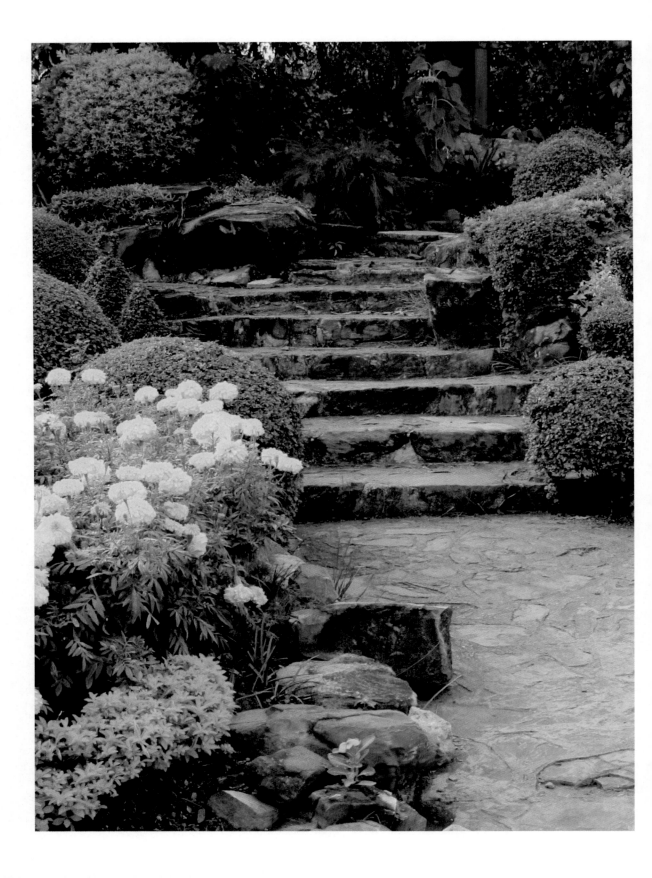

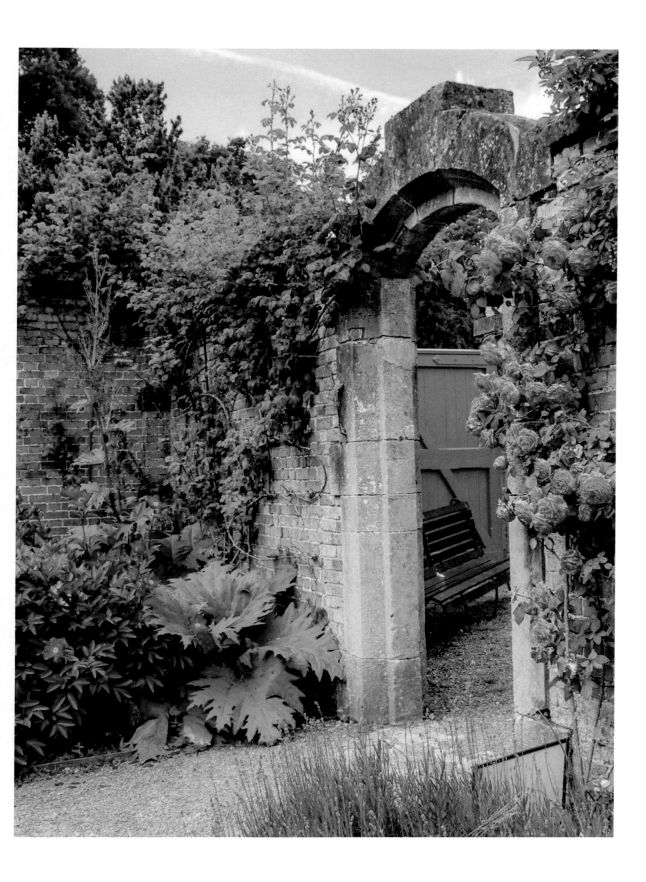

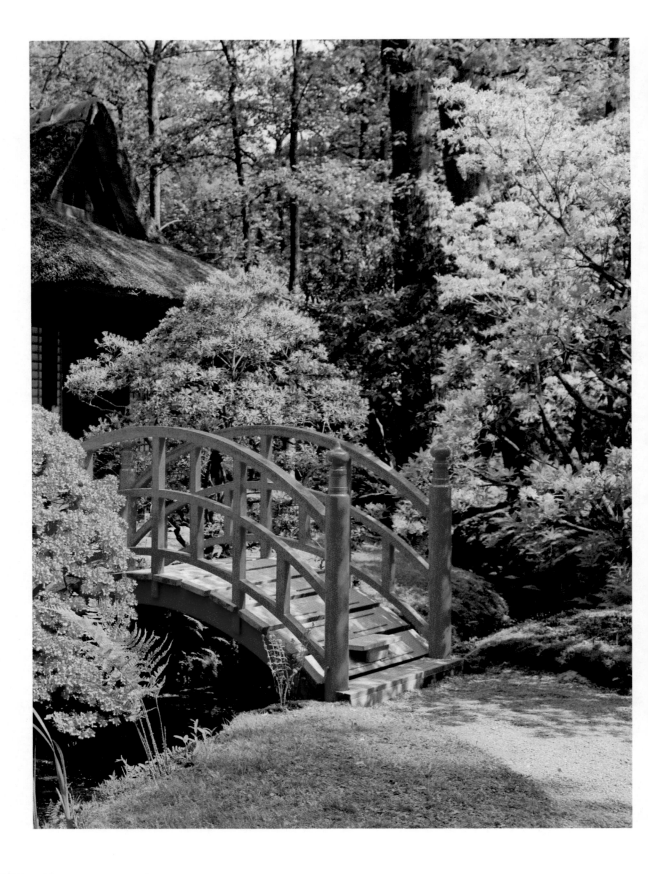

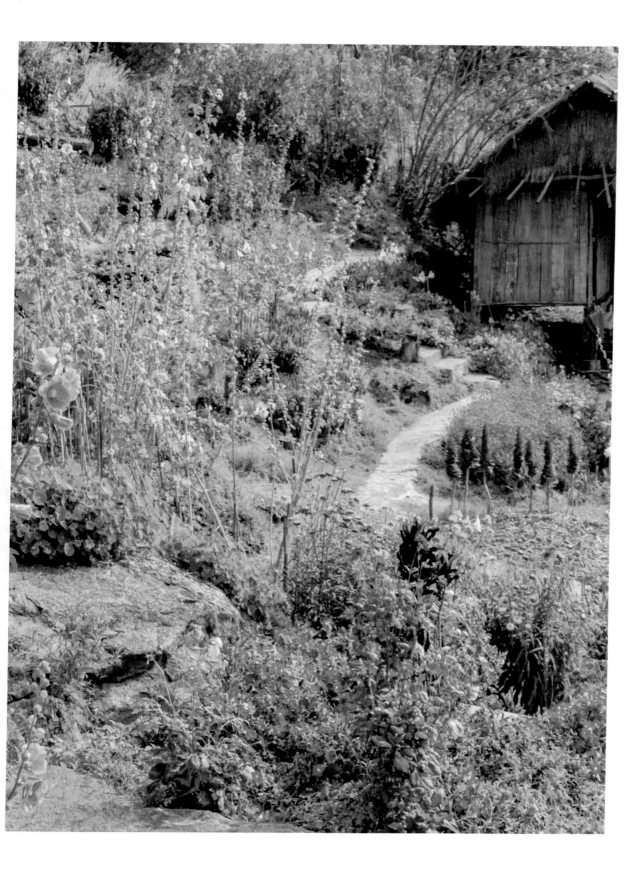

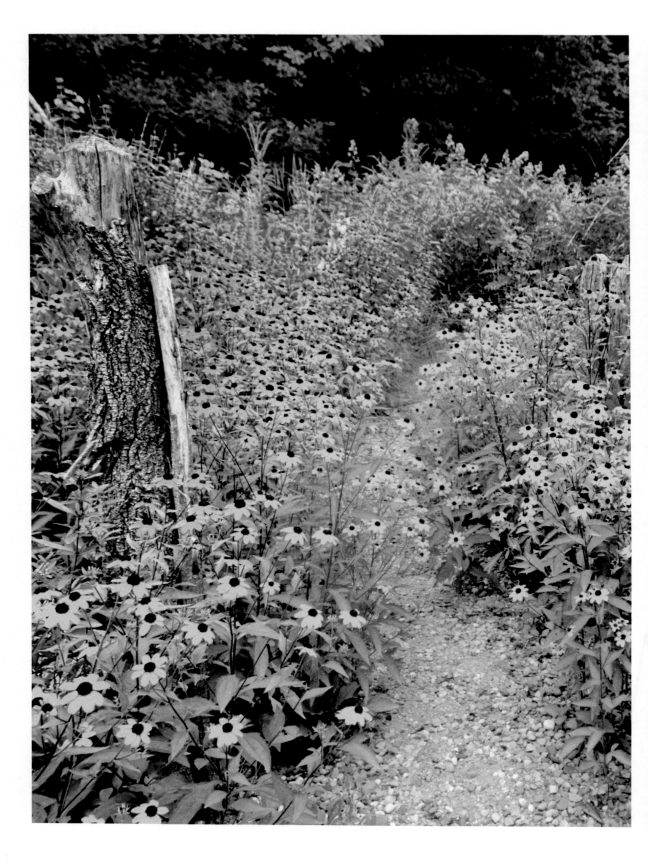

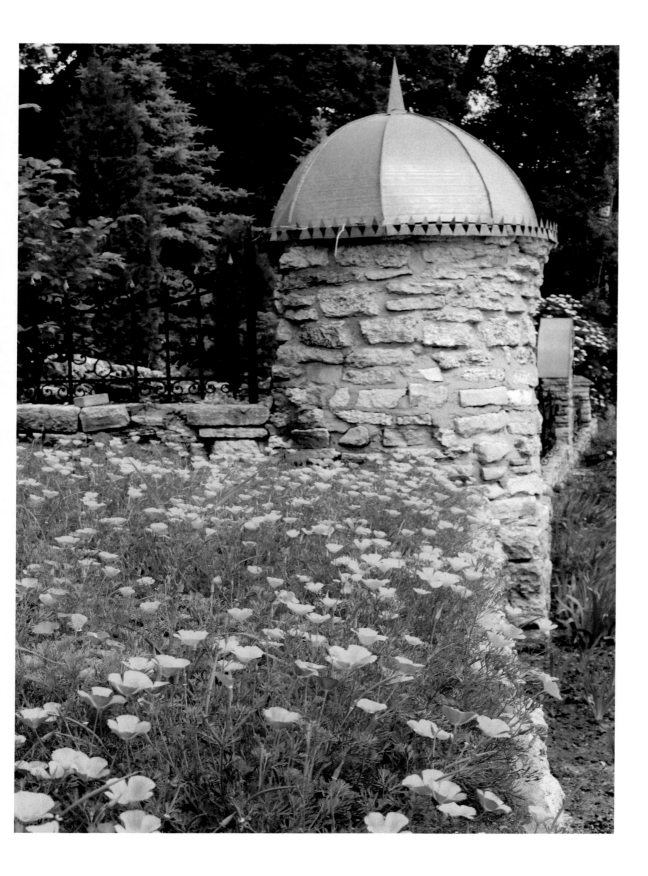

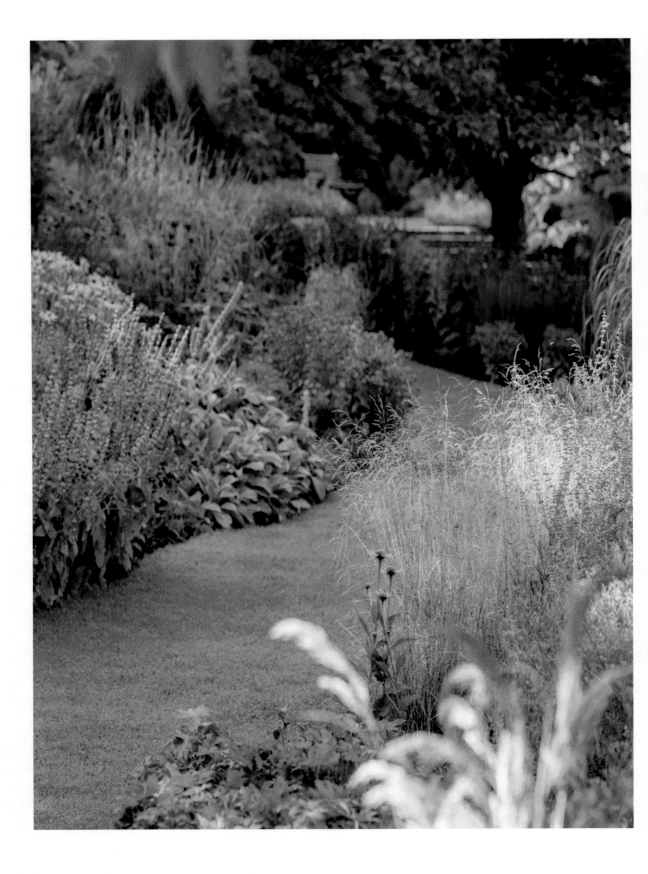

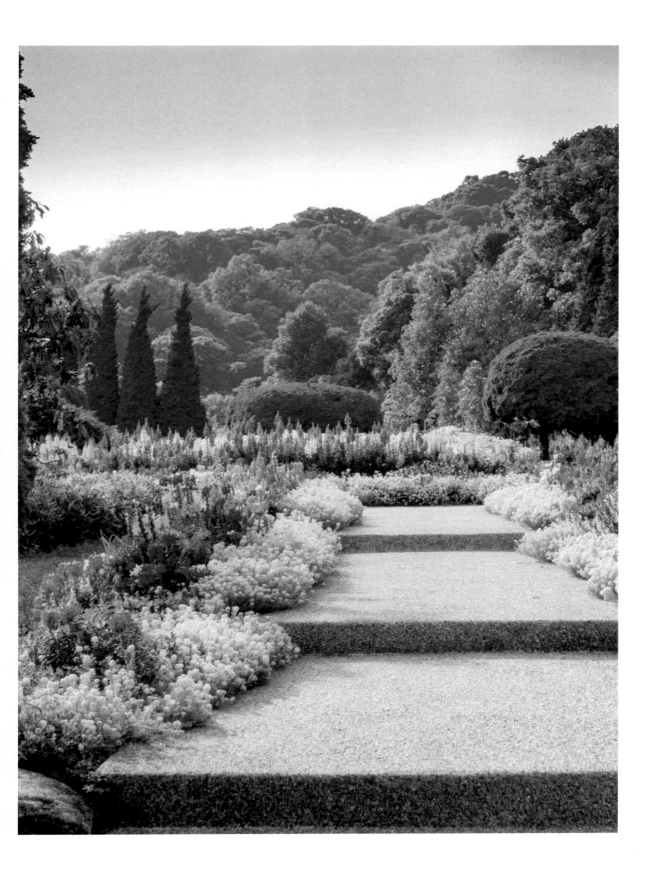

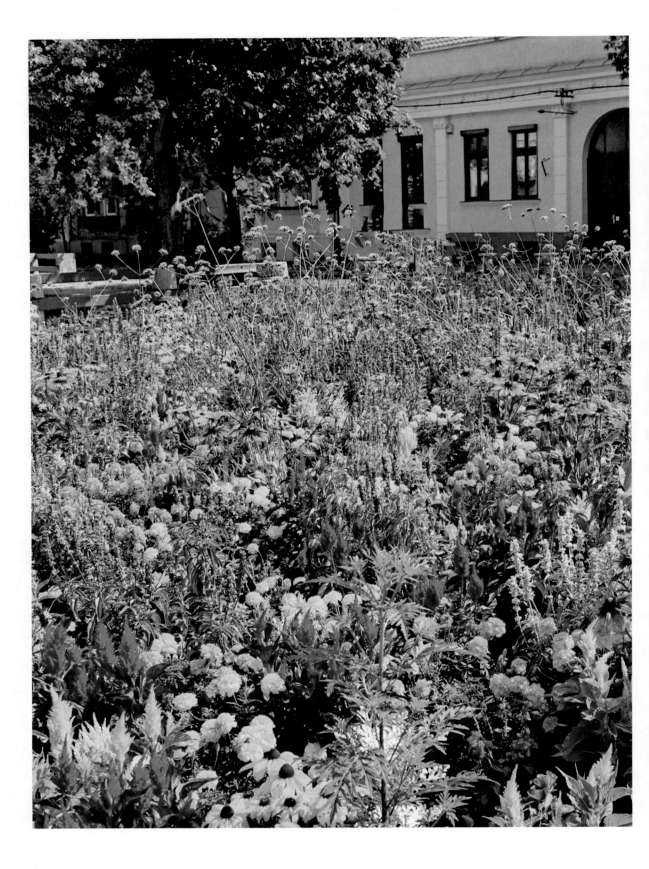

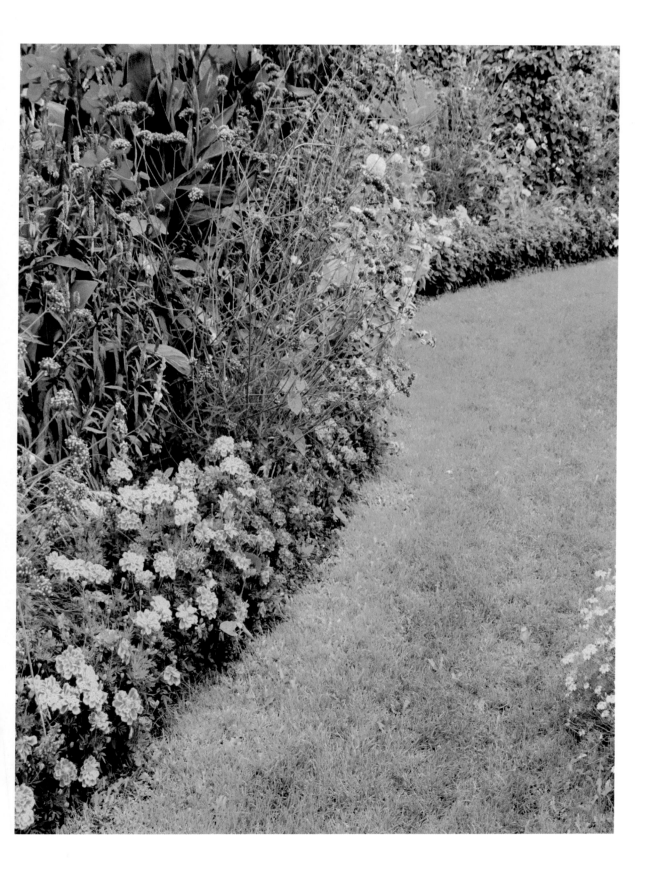

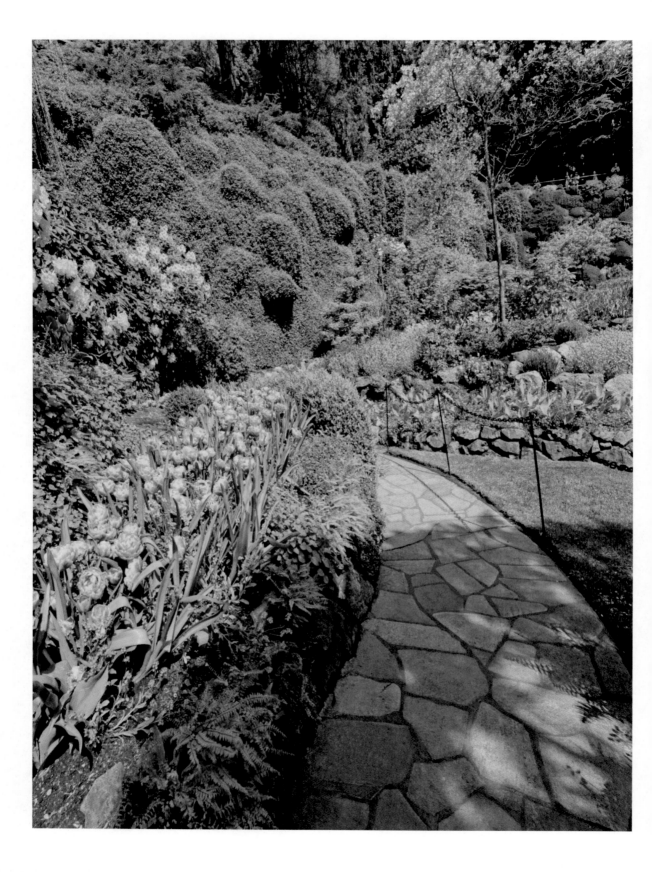

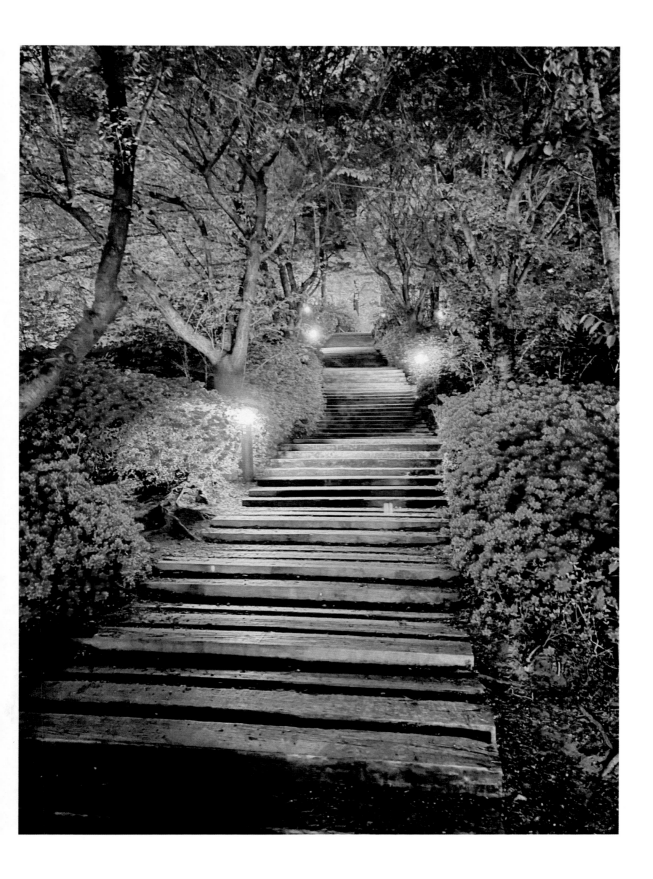

Thank you

Thanks for your interest in our books.

Please consider purchasing our other books
available now at Amazon.com.

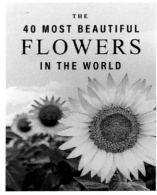
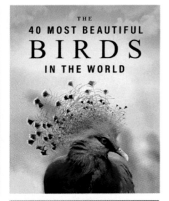
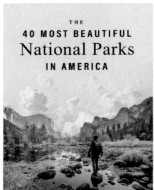
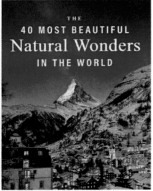

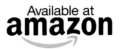

(Just search for "Blue Clover Books" on Amazon.)

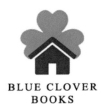

Made in the USA
Middletown, DE
28 March 2024

52227053R00024